What they're saying about
KNOW YOUR ENEMY: Taking the Fight to Cancer

"It was my privilege to take care of Mrs. Antonicelli. I think it is fantastic that this book is a product of Frank's experiences and can now help other families. It is an excellent guide through the complicated path of cancer—for both the patient and their family."

— *Ruchi Dash, MD*

"The comfortable layout in this book will have you easily going from cover to cover in only a few sittings. The information Frank presents would have been invaluable during the many years of my young daughter's leukemia struggles while I was a single mother raising two other children."

— *Deborah Maguire*

"We hear the word cancer and we enter a new and frightening world. We reach for our faith, the support of our family and friends, and another vital ally—knowledge about the path to come. Mr. Antonicelli has written a terrific book that helps us find that path. Lots of good information and advice and encouragement fill its pages."

— *Kathryn Peroutka, MD*

"As an oncologist who lost his own father to cancer, I truly believe this book is a much needed resource that will help to better inform and empower all of our patients and their families."

— *Paul Y. Song, MD*

"Frank's willingness to openly share his family's struggle with cancer is to your benefit. You'll find yourself saying, 'Me too. That's exactly what I'm feeling,' quite often. If this book was available when my brother successfully fought stomach cancer, ten years ago, it would have made things much easier for our family."

— *Pete Weaver*

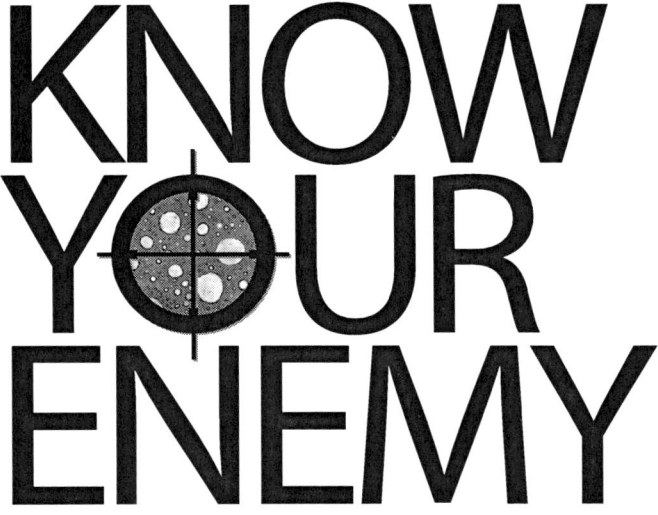

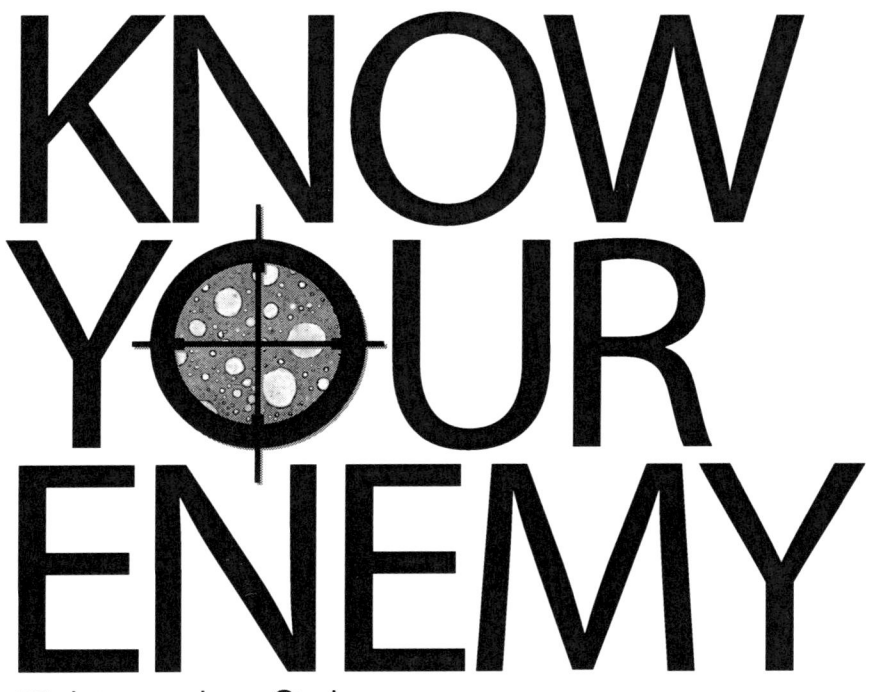

KNOW YOUR ENEMY

Taking the fight to cancer

Frank Antonicelli

Copyright © 2016 Frank Antonicelli
All rights reserved
First Edition

PAGE PUBLISHING, INC.
New York, NY

First originally published by Page Publishing, Inc. 2016
Cover art designed by 206 Design 2015

ISBN 978-1-68213-017-9 (pbk)
ISBN 978-1-68213-018-6 (digital)
ISBN 978-1-68289-749-2 (hardcover)

Printed in the United States of America

*"There are those who look at things the
way they are, and ask why…
I dream of things that never were,
and ask why not."*

—Robert F. Kennedy

Disclaimer

The information in this book is true and complete to the best of our knowledge. This book is intended only as an informative guide for those wishing to know more about health issues. In no way is this book intended to replace, countermand, or conflict the advice given to you by your own physician. The ultimate decision concerning care should be made between you and your doctor. We strongly recommend you follow his or her advice. Information in this book is general and offered with no guarantees on the part of the author. The author and publisher declaim all liability in connection with the use of this book.

CONTENTS

Foreword by Dr. Matthew Mumber 13

Introduction: The Word..15

Chapter 1: Gather Your Troops 21

Chapter 2: Leading the Charge..30

Chapter 3: Know Your Enemy 38

Chapter 4: The Battle Plan 48

Chapter 5: The Soul of Battle...57

Chapter 6: Timing Is Everything 65

Chapter 7: Gathering Intel 71

Chapter 8: The Power of Faith 80

Chapter 9: Winning Is a Mindset 85

Chapter 10: I'm Still Standing..91

Epilogue: Last Words..97

Acknowledgments 103

DEDICATION

This book is dedicated to a special group of individuals I view as the true warriors in our society today, not to be confused with so-called warrior athletes, labeled as such by exhibiting their superior talents on the field of play. The individuals I am referring to are engaged in a daily struggle against a formidable health opponent—cancer. These modern-day warriors are not playing a kids' game; they are adults and children, patients and caregivers, and medical professionals faced with the daunting task of battling a cowardly and menacing enemy—cancer—day in and day out, with everything they can muster.

They are the chemotherapy patients on a cocktail so strong they have little energy to get out of bed in the morning—or the radiation patients that suffer treatment side effects, such as severe joint or nerve pain or burning skin. Add to these difficulties the responsibilities of raising a family or maintaining a career, and now you're talking about a Herculean effort just to make it through the day. They are the caregivers whose world becomes turned upside down and then fixated on battling this enemy when a loved one is confronted with a cancer diagnosis. Last, but not least, they are the medical professionals on the front lines caring for, supporting, and consoling patients and family members in their greatest time of need.

My mother, Maxine, and my wife, Alyson, were two very strong and determined women that epitomize what it means to be a modern-day-warrior cancer patient. Both were blind-sided with the news of a cancer diagnosis, yet they confronted this health challenge with a quiet calm and confidence. They did not shy away from these health challenges, and as the subtitle of this book states, they took the fight to cancer!

Do you have someone in your life that has exhibited extraordinary strength of character in this battle against the enemy? If so, have you told this person that he (or she) is your hero? If not, what are you waiting for?

To my mother, Maxine R. Antonicelli; my wife, Alyson C. Antonicelli; my little buddy, Derek Johnson #223 (son of Tina and Scott Johnson); my personal friend and neighbor, Stephen B. Wagoner; and all those who are engaged against the enemy—cancer—this book is dedicated to you, for you are true warriors, gladiators in the arena of life.

Frank Antonicelli
New Cumberland, Pennsylvania
November 2015

THE MAN IN THE ARENA

Excerpt from Theodore Roosevelt's speech
"Citizenship in a Republic"
Delivered at the Sorbonne in Paris, France, on April 23, 1910

"It is not the critic who counts; not the man who points out how the strong man stumbles, or where the doer of deeds could have done them better. The credit belongs to the man who is actually in the arena, whose face is marred by dust and sweat and blood; who strives valiantly; who errs, who comes short again and again, because there is no effort without error and shortcoming; but who does actually strive to do the deeds; who knows great enthusiasms, the great devotions; who spends himself in a worthy cause; who at the best knows in the end the triumph of high achievement, and who at the worst, if he fails, at least fails while daring greatly, so that his place shall never be with those cold and timid souls who neither know victory nor defeat."

FOREWORD BY
DR. MATTHEW MUMBER

Q: What do a biblical author of Proverbs, the rock band Aerosmith, and Vince Lombardi have in common?
A: They all offer insight on the life path of caring and cancer.

If you find this a bit of a stretch, then the book *Know Your Enemy* will offer you some surprises, a few tears, and a load of inspiration. This book provides accurate information concerning the cancer journey and is a wonderful supplemental tool for those undergoing cancer treatment and their families.

I have been fortunate to be involved in the journeys of tens of thousands of cancer patients and their loved ones over the past twenty years of my practice as a radiation oncologist. Over that time, I have never met any two individuals that are exactly alike. My work focuses on an approach to medicine that includes all participants in the process and engages them at all levels of their being and experience. It is through a focus on inclusion that we move forward and grow: both/and instead of either/or.

An integrative approach to cancer care includes all participants—patient, family members, doctors, other care providers, and community members. It addresses each of these players at all levels of their being: mind, body, and spirit.

It looks through all of these levels aware of the lenses through which we see life—the perspectives of our individual self, our cultural background, and the natural world in which we live. This broad approach allows all parts of ourselves to be experienced and become an avenue through which to explore healing. Everything belongs.

True healing dives deep and moves beyond a superficial skimming along the surface of our lives. In this frame of mind, deep speaks to deep, and any life event can become a source of inspiration to guide us along on the path of transformation—the path of seeing things with new eyes like an innocent child. All of us have a calling, and we can be lit up from both within and without. This guidance will always come to those willing to stop, look, and listen.

It is said that God comes to each of us disguised as our life. We have the opportunity to listen to the soundtrack of our life in a way that has never been done before in the infinity of existence. Our unique life is a tremendous gift, and we open up the present by the powerful yet simple will to listen, with mercy and awareness to whatever comes up without trying to fix it. It can be done. Frank Antonicelli offers written proof that it is possible to follow the path of transformation that is often brought on by great love and great suffering.

In *Know Your Enemy*, Frank listens to his life. In so doing, inspiration comes from everywhere and from nowhere. He encounters God. God is in the living and in the dying. God is in the enemy and in the friend.

Read this book as proof that you too can encounter life through whatever struggles and joys that you may face. Dive deep, if only for a moment each day, and taste your one-of-a-kind, never-to-be-repeated life.

Dr. Matthew Mumber is an award-winning board-certified radiation oncologist and codirector of the MD Ambassador Program and Integrative Oncology Program at Harbin Clinic in Rome, Georgia. Dr. Mumber is coauthor of **Sustainable Wellness: An Integrative Approach to Transform Your Mind, Body, and Spirit**. *He gives talks, leads workshops, and writes extensively on integrative approaches to oncology, health, and wellness. Dr. Mumber is the founder of the nonprofit organization Cancer Navigators, Inc.*

INTRODUCTION

THE WORD

"We all have a fear of the unknown. What one does with that fear will make all the difference in the world."

—Lillian Russell

When cancer invades your life, it doesn't just politely knock on your door, it breaks the door down. It is only after you pick yourself up and dust yourself off, that you realize you are in a battle against a formidable adversary.

Maxine

In the case of my family, the enemy came without warning. It was a holiday weekend—Labor Day 2011. In fact, there may have been warning signs, but if there were, not one of us ever saw them. That's how it is with this enemy; he sneaks up on you when you're not looking. Then, you have to retrace your steps to figure out how you missed the signs.

What seemed to "happen so fast" had actually begun six months earlier when my mother, Maxine (Max), began complaining to us of minor back pain. As the holiday weekend progressed, she began to lose feeling in her legs. By the time she woke up Monday morning, she was unable to stand on her own.

From this point on, the details are hazy. I know that we called an ambulance and rushed Max to the Harrisburg Hospital emergency room. Other members of our family and some of my mother's close friends soon joined us.

I remember that the ER doctor informed us she would be running a series of tests to determine what was causing Max's paralysis. After that, time passed slowly—I realized later that what seemed like an eternity had only been ninety minutes. The ER doctor called us back into Max's makeshift hospital room. Max lay on the bed, motionless, a trace of fear in her eyes, all of us gathered around her.

When the doctor spoke, she was standing right next to me, but it sounded as if she were speaking from the other end of a long hallway. "I'm sorry to have to tell you that the results of the scan show a sizeable growth in Maxine's right upper lung. The tumor, which appears to be cancerous, is pushing against her spinal cord and this is most likely the cause of Max's current paralysis." Looking back, we realized that this tumor had been gradually causing Max greater pain over the last six months.

The minute that I heard the word "cancer," my body immediately went numb. The room and my surroundings became eerily quiet, and everything appeared to be happening in slow motion. I felt oddly distanced from myself, as if I were watching a movie about some other family. When the world started coming back, I could hear the familiar voices of family members and the ER doctor discussing my mom's condition. This was no movie—it was real. I knew at that moment that my life would never be the same. Something ugly and menacing had entered my life without my permission. I would have to face it, but at that moment, I had no idea how I would.

Alyson

It was only seven months after Max's diagnosis when I found myself sitting in a doctor's office at the Milton S. Hershey Medical Center in Hershey, Pennsylvania. I remember thinking to myself, *If I never see another doctor's office, it would be just fine with me.* Alyson sat next to me, her brown eyes staring straight ahead, her hands folded in her lap.

Once again, we were waiting for a diagnosis—this time, the biopsy results from a growth found in Alyson's reproductive system. For days, we had told each other the best, but now we silently prepared ourselves for the worst.

Alyson's oncologist and his assistant appeared, and suddenly I felt a chill in the room. The enemy was back. "I'm sorry to have to tell you this, but unfortunately, the lesion has turned out to be a squamous cell carcinoma, which means we will have to remove it immediately."

Perhaps you are thinking as you read this that the news of my wife's cancer diagnosis should have made me a candidate for a rubber room and a little red rubber ball. Here I had just gone through months of battling this monstrous disease with my mother, and now I was being asked to step up again and resume the fight with my wife. You might think this, but you would be wrong.

I can honestly say that, this time, hearing the word "cancer" gave me an immediate surge of energy and motivation and a real sense of purpose. Instead of becoming distanced from my body, I felt more focused than I had ever been. Thoughts entered my brain, one after the other, in rapid succession. One thought was *Okay, you know the drill*. I did. I knew exactly what I had to do, and that knowledge was power.

How This Book Came About

As you can probably tell by now, I'm not one to pout or complain about my lot in life. We had been struck a low blow, but I was fighting back to the best of my ability. However, one day, I sat in my living room, thinking about all we'd been through. I thought about how tough it had been, going through cancer for the first time. *Damn*, I thought, *this is hell and no one should have to go through this experience.*

Winston Churchill said, *"If you are going through hell, keep going,"* and that is how I'm wired. Suddenly, it came to me that there was something I could actually do about it—something beyond waging our own battles with the enemy. By writing about our experiences, perhaps I could help others going through cancer for the first time. I thought if I could help just one person battling this ruthless enemy, my efforts would be worth it.

The result of that "aha" moment is the book you now hold in your hands. It is an outgrowth of days of learning, planning, researching, thinking, and finally, acting. It is based largely upon the ideas that supported me throughout our battles with the enemy—the teachings of the great Chinese philosopher Sun Tzu. Sun Tzu's words have always been inspirational to me, and I will have much more to say about his writings and teachings later on in the book, but for now, here are the lines from Sun Tzu's "Warrior Rules" that inspired this book's title:

> *If you know your enemy and yourself, you need not fear the results of a hundred battles.*

It is my hope that this book will help you go from being "knocked down" by the enemy to combat mode. With the great "warrior rules" planted firmly in your head, I hope you will respond to cancer with a "battle plan" of your own. I want you to get to know your specific cancer and type better than it knows you or your loved one. Acquire the knowledge you need to beat cancer at its own game. Gather the confidence that comes from making informed decisions on the battlefield. Above all, *know your enemy.*

Like our battles, your battle against cancer may encompass a wide range of emotions. The highs may carry you through for days, until a time comes that you feel you can't go on—a time when, as a friend said to me, "you get to the point where you are tired of being tired." I hope this book will be a comfort to you and that it inspires you to go the distance. Remember, you are not alone. There are countless professionals and organizations there to help you each step of the way; many of them are listed in the pages of this book.

If, like me, you are waging this battle against the enemy on behalf of someone you love, all the more reason to be armed and ready. I promise you this health challenge you face is like no other. You must acquire the knowledge to go toe-to-toe with this enemy and the confidence to know that you are making informed decisions at every step in your journey.

Regardless of your needs—whether it's you who has cancer or someone you love—I urge you to keep the words of Sun Tzu in your back pocket: *"If you know your enemy and yourself, you need not fear the results of a hundred battles."* Time is of the essence, and this enemy waits for no one. Carpe diem.

Final Thoughts: The Word

Regardless of your initial state of mind when you first hear "the word" (cancer), it's important to remember that you've got to get yourself in gear as quickly as possible.

Remember

- There is no right way to feel or act when you first learn of a cancer diagnosis.
- Take comfort in knowing that there are countless professionals and organizations dedicated to helping you battle this enemy.

"Life is ten percent what happens to you and ninety percent how you respond to it."

—Lou Holtz

CHAPTER 1

GATHER YOUR TROOPS

"A single arrow is easily broken but not ten in a bundle."
—Japanese proverb

The battle begins: it's you versus the enemy. Cancer has an arsenal of weapons at its disposal, including the element of surprise, a history of brutality, and the ability to disguise itself to evade detection. As I mentioned earlier, cancer's initial assault can be overwhelming and immediately put you in a defensive posture, as it attacks your physical, mental, emotional, and financial well-being. Cancer is, simply put, a test of your strength and will. How do you go up against such a shape-shifting monster?

One thing I can tell you: first, gather your troops! Think of the famous battles throughout history, from the Alamo to Gettysburg. In every instance of resounding success, a strong military leader was surrounded by loyal troops. To successfully blunt an initial attack and respond with an equally forceful counter-offensive, you must first realize the importance of working as a team, as there is strength in numbers. Remember the scene from *Braveheart* when Mel Gibson, as Scottish-rebel William Wallace, charged across the field, rallying his men to fight for their liberty and not to yield? The opposing side was so taken off guard by the force of their onslaught that they lost the battle and, ultimately, the war.

As our family battled the enemy, we were grateful to have the support of family members and friends, especially as treatment got under way and it became more difficult to handle all the details ourselves. Get all the help you need from anyone and everyone who offers it, and for as long as you need it. Cancer is brutal. No matter your strength, when a helping hand reaches out—take it! As Inspector Harry Callahan ("Dirty Harry") famously quipped in the film *Magnum Force,* "A man has got to know his limitations."

I realize that letting people in can be a challenge, especially if you're the type that is usually independent, self-sufficient, or private by nature. If you are used to going it alone, then you may have trouble accepting kind offers from friends and family members. But I promise you that cancer is like no other enemy you have ever faced. Even if all you do is accept modest amounts of support, you will definitely want some help as your battle with this enemy intensifies.

Finding Your Foot Soldiers

If you have a big support group, as I luckily do, then family members and friends may want to play a key role in your battle against cancer. If you want this assistance to be useful and to come how and when you need it, then you will have to know who the best people are for the tasks at hand. However, when family members or friends are unable to help for one reason or another, it is important that you be sensitive to their availability and capability.

Regarding Max's and Alyson's battles with cancer, we initially thought that we, the family members, were the "generals" controlling the battle. This approach evoked anxiety, stress, and tension for all of us, as we later came to realize that we were out of step with the real generals, Max and Alyson. We learned that we would have to rein ourselves in and stay in the moment to be in sync with Max's and Alyson's physical, emotional, and mental energies. This enlightened approach allowed us to delegate tasks to our troops in a more efficient manner. Those who couldn't help directly were always kept in the loop (more later on exactly how we accomplished this).

You may find your best troops among friends or family. Throughout our long battle with the enemy, we counted on not only our friends but also our family members, and used their generosity and support in much the same way. Whether friends or family, both are there for you because they care about you and want to help you through a difficult time. They just want you to let them know how and when they can help.

My advice is to take a direct approach, right from the start. Once you have identified the troops you can trust, make sure they have the time and energy to be involved for the duration of the battle. Try to identify alternative ways to participate for all those interested, based on their time and ability.

As the battle becomes more complicated, you will need to assign troops who can act as gatekeepers. Believe me when I say you won't have the time, energy, or patience to communicate directly with everyone in your circle via e-mail, text, or phone. Getting the word out through your gatekeepers prevents misunderstandings and hurt feelings, the last thing you want during a time when you need every bit of support you can get.

Get Organized

When the enemy makes the first appearance, you will have to reach beyond your fear and panic and take charge. This is the hardest part but it's important, as it forms the basis of what will become an overall strategy. Get as organized as possible at this time, as it will help you later on as treatment intensifies.

To get started, hold an initial "health intelligence briefing" for all concerned. Here, you will dispense important information to all who have offered their help, directly or indirectly. First, lay out the medical situation, explaining the diagnosis and likely course of treatment. Discuss practical needs like driving to doctor visits or preparing meals. Getting organized is the basis of any good battle plan, and in this case, it has another benefit: it helps everyone feel less powerless.

At your first health intelligence briefing, encourage your troops to come up with a plan of action for keeping everyone informed. As you move along, it's important to have each person in the loop so you can make use of whatever help is offered. Your supporters may want to set up a "phone chain." Or they may do it the modern way, using Facebook or Twitter, or even establishing a special website where information can be relayed. CaringBridge.com is one such site that helps families stay connected during a health event.

I should also mention that it is okay to keep some information private. Don't feel that just because you have established a network, you have to share every bit of information. Even your trusted troops don't need to know every detail—only what you wish to share. This is your health issue, and you get to choose how much information is disseminated and to whom. Just do your best not to offend, and try to make use of any help that is offered. Remember that not allowing someone to contribute to the process may be felt as a rejection or lack of appreciation for what is essentially a gesture of loving-kindness.

During this preplanning phase, you and your troops will want to figure out what type of help is most needed—driving to doctors' appointments, preparing meals, babysitting for children, or caring for pets—any help that may support you during the treatment should be on the list. If your extended friends and family members are anything like ours were, you can anticipate many generous offers to help and support you in your battle against this enemy. Remember to keep their specific interests in mind and to figure out which people can be most useful and in what capacity. It's important not to overlook anyone's good intentions.

This is an appropriate time to mention that if you have friends or family members in the medical field, don't hesitate to call on them as additional medical experts or specialists. They know your family and can be trusted to provide honest answers during this difficult time. Of course, you'll have to respect their boundaries and time constraints.

The Healing Power of Love

Deepak Chopra has written, "The use of love is to heal. When it flows without effort from the depth of the self, love creates health." I believe this to be true, as I've seen the power of love in action. In fact, I believe love may be the single greatest weapon in your treatment arsenal. Why? *Because love is a foreign concept to cancer.* The love you receive from those who really care about you has the potential to bring this enemy to its knees.

During the early days of Max's and Alyson's treatments, I had tunnel vision. I was so focused on cancer that I all but ignored my friends, and my conversations with them were few and far between. As time went on, I welcomed the opportunity to talk about something other than cancer. When I could, I spent time chatting with them about their own lives and caught up with other family news. Just having a shoulder to lean on provided a welcome escape from my daily skirmishes with this enemy.

Taking a break from the enemy can be difficult at first. You may feel that your entire being is engaged in a continuous, knockdown, drag-out battle. However, if you are able to break out of the single-minded state of being, these breaks can provide you with a much-needed respite. Taking a mental vacation from cancer, and getting a hug from a friend, is as important to your battle against the enemy as any prescription a doctor might write. *Remember, love heals.*

Another type of loving support may come to you during this time from your four-legged friends—the pet(s) that know you and love you unconditionally and seem to sense that you need them now more than ever. During Alyson's battle with cancer, we both relied heavily on our wonderful Siamese cat, Simon. We jokingly referred to him as her "comfort cat" because he literally took on the lead role as Alyson's personal protector. Simon's actions reinforced my belief that the family pet instinctively senses our full range of human emotions. Whether or not you have a "Simon" in your life, I encourage you to find an animal to pet, lie on your lap, or just hang out with you for a while. I promise it will make you feel better and lighten the overall mood for your family.

Final Thoughts: Gather Your Troops

There is no doubt that battling this enemy requires all the support you can get, whether it is from family members, close friends, or pets.

Remember

- People want to help—let them know what kind of help is needed.
- Delegate some responsibility to your "troops."
- You are not alone; take the help that is offered.

"The nice thing about teamwork is that you always have others on your side."

—Margaret Carty

During what turned out to be one of the most grueling periods in my life, I was blessed with the support and love of friends and family members. Their genuine acts of kindness and compassion reinforced my belief in the goodness of others and the notion of having a greater purpose in life. One night, while reflecting upon these special acts of love and kindness, I wrote the following poem to express my gratitude to this special group of individuals:

The Chosen Few

When a life-changing event rocks your world to the core,
Who will pick you up, as you rise from the floor?
Consider yourself blessed, if your earthly sphere includes
A special band of brothers, I refer to as The Chosen Few.
No obstacle is too great, for this brotherhood to overcome.
And no quarter will they cede until the final battle is won.
Of whom do I speak? Who are these chosen few?
They are a special band of brothers, and one of them is you.
So in these words, I thank you, more than you will ever know.
And, if the need shall one day arise, I, too, will stand with you.

Notes

Notes

CHAPTER 2

LEADING THE CHARGE

"You will find peace not by trying to escape your problems, but by confronting them courageously. You will find peace not in denial, but in victory."

—J. Donald Walters

Just as no battle can be fought or won alone, every great counteroffensive requires an unwavering leader—one who is centered and confident enough to command his troops and lead the charge against the enemy. Sun Tzu captured this eloquent description of true leadership in battle in these two lines from *The Art of War*:

*Move swift as the wind and closely-formed as wood.
Attack like the fire and be still as the mountain.*

What did Sun Tzu mean when he wrote that a leader must be "swift," but also held together like "wood"? How is it possible to attack "like the fire" yet "be still as the mountain"? Perhaps Sun Tzu was referring to the balance that arises from being all things at once, and the knowledge and power that come from inner peace. He understood that when we carry the burden of insecurity or fear, fueled by memories of our past failures, we are as likely to be defeated by our own impulses as by the enemy. Sun Tzu did not live in modern times, but what he understood about coming to terms with the enemy holds true today: *When we enter the challenge as whole and balanced individuals, we are invincible.*

As you enter your battle against cancer, you must first restore physical and mental wholeness. You must become aware of and aggressively eliminate any emotional issues that might be fueling the enemy's assault. This means banishing circumstances or situations that may be creating unnecessary stress, tension, or anxiety. With these distractions removed, you become as "swift as the wind" and as "still as the mountain." You are ready for the enemy.

Assessing Stress

Whether or not cancer begins in the body as a response to stress remains to be proven. But I believe, as Don Henley writes in "The Heart of the Matter":

> *You better put it behind you; cause life goes on*
> *You keep carryin' that anger, it'll eat you up inside baby.*

So why does the enemy find its way to some of us and not others? And how do you face the possibility that you may have been your own worst enemy? For medical science, the jury is still out on this debate about whether stress causes cancer. But it is clear, we would all do well to release any stress in our bodies by bringing our problems closer to the surface where we can resolve and defeat them.

If you or someone you love has already been diagnosed with cancer, then it pays to ask: What types of self-defeating behaviors were brought to the battlefield? What types of situations or circumstances could be fueling this enemy? There may be family, career, relationship, and/or financial issues that are impacting your daily life. Perhaps certain life choices you made long ago are affecting you to this day. These issues, over time, can take a huge physical and mental toll on the human body.

It is time to let them go. In this battle of and for life, you must be centered and still—the strongest that you have ever been. If there are emotional burdens weighing your life down, you must develop a plan to release them. This enemy thrives on weakness, so you must show strength. Your swiftness and stillness will surprise the enemy.

Here's one more thing to consider: when you think about things that might be causing stress, don't just look at what is happening right at this moment. All human emotion has a half-life. Perhaps there was a divorce five years ago, but the trauma of that event is still gnawing, deep inside. Or there might be the experience of the death of a loved one without ever completing the grieving process. If that's the case, this needs to be done right away so that life can move on. To do battle with this enemy, there must be peace with the past.

Once you identify the root cause(s) of any issues, it may be helpful to discuss them with a therapist, spiritual advisor, friend, or family member. Getting these issues out in the open might make it easier to release them. It might also be helpful during this time to begin some type of spiritual or physical discipline, such as yoga or meditation, to restore peace and balance to your life. I encourage you to try to incorporate at least one of the following disciplines to help in this time of need.

Meditation and Prayer

The power of meditation and prayer has been well documented as a way to reduce stress, tension, and anxiety. Meditation or prayer allows individuals to clear their mind, similar to pushing a mental reset button each day. The focus can then be directed toward positive thoughts and visual images to harness the healing power of the mind and body. Many cancer treatment centers recognize the value of meditation for their patients. At Massachusetts General Hospital, a rooftop "healing garden" offers patients and their families a quiet place to take a break from treatment, amidst tropical plants and the soothing sounds of flowing water.

During Max's battle, she was able to find great strength and comfort in her faith and the power of prayer. Her favorite scripture, which we displayed in her room, says*: "Trust in the Lord with all your heart and lean not on your own understanding; in all your ways acknowledge him, and he will direct your paths." (Proverbs 3:5–6)* Max also shared a special bond with her pastor that grew even stronger when he later learned he would have to battle this enemy as well. Through their Bible discussions, both found an inner peace that provided great support.

Positive Thoughts and Visualization Techniques

Many athletes use positive thoughts and imagery to focus and encourage them on the field. This positive mental framework is a motivational force that lifts spirit and focus throughout the game. To assist patients at various stages of recovery, positive thoughts and visualization techniques are frequently combined with a meditation and prayer exercise as a way to enhance the healing power of the mind and body. These techniques help release unwanted thoughts and emotions by framing positive thoughts and images for the patient to focus on.

During Max's and Alyson's treatments, we used some of these techniques. In Max's case, we charted and made a huge deal about each gain she made during physical therapy. Alyson created her own positive image: the swimsuit she had worn during her last Masters swim-team practice. She kept it hanging on a hook in the bathroom throughout her treatment. She was not going to let this enemy change her workout routine—hanging her wet suit in the bathroom to dry for the next practice—and was already envisioning herself back in the pool doing what she loved to do: swim 50s.

Physical Fitness and Exercise

Any exercise, be it cardiovascular training or muscle strength or flexibility training, can provide you with an opportunity to increase your energy and endurance levels—critical tools to have in your arsenal when battling cancer. Studies have shown that exercise releases endorphins in the brain, providing great therapeutic effects and a "natural high" that may help you conquer fear, self-doubt, and other limitations. Exercise was a big part of both Max's and Alyson's treatment programs. As stated earlier, Max was involved in intensive physical and occupational therapies. Alyson followed an individualized program developed by the Block Center that focused on increasing her endurance and overall strength to battle this enemy.

Diet, Nutrition, and Supplements

The body undergoing cancer treatment needs the right kind of fuel to enable it to withstand the rigors of a traditional cancer treatment regimen. If available, I encourage you to work with a nutritionist to find the right balance of vitamins, minerals, nutrients, and when required, supplements. Both Max and Alyson relied on a nutritionist to develop a comprehensive dietary program tailored to their individual needs.

Yoga

A yoga workout can provide both a mental and physical reset, clearing the mind and body of unproductive stress and anxiety that have built up as a result of daily living. Yoga can be used in combination with meditation, prayer, positive thinking, and visualization to enhance the natural healing processes of the mind and body, including those supporting your fight against the enemy.

Laughter and Humor

The power of laughter has been documented to have special healing powers. No matter how grim things looked, it's important to make laughter a part of your day. Max loved *The Carol Burnett Show*. During her hospital stay, we bought her several DVDs of the show and watched them with her every day. It was amazing how this one act not only lightened the mood for Max but also provided a much-needed escape for family, friends, and even the hospital staff.

Listening to Music

Like laughter, the power of music has also been well documented. Whether it's a relaxing tune on the radio to listen to, or the comforting lyrics of a song from your youth, music presents yet another way for you to alter mood and energy levels and provide a positive distraction as you fight against cancer. Music can have a direct medical benefit. According to the Mayo Clinic, music can actually reduce physical pain and counteract depression. So, whether you crank up Led Zeppelin or tune into some Bach, make music a part of the daily regimen and watch the enemy recede into the background. Music provided joy and relaxation for our family, as well as a therapeutic escape from the burdens of battle.

Final Thoughts: Leading the Charge

To defeat this enemy successfully, you must strive to eliminate any emotional issues that may be fueling the enemy's assault. This means eliminating unhealthy relationships or situations that may be creating unnecessary stress, tension, or anxiety.

Remember

- You cannot defeat this enemy unless you are both "swift" and "still."
- You must identify and release current issues and emotional baggage.
- Use everything in your arsenal to eliminate stress and anxiety.

"The task of the leader is to get his people from where they are to where they have not been."

—Henry Kissinger

Notes

Notes

CHAPTER 3

KNOW YOUR ENEMY

"Data is meaningless, information is knowledge, and knowledge is power."
—James McGee and Laurence Prusak

To a cancer patient or family member, hearing a doctor discuss a cancer diagnosis or treatment in "med-speak," as I call it, is like hearing someone talking in a foreign language. Med-speak refers to the unique vocabulary the medical oncology community uses to define and discuss common cancer terms with patients and family members. You must get up to speed quickly and become fluent in med-speak because, for this journey, it will become your second language.

The information provided in this chapter will help you to become familiar with common cancer terminology or "med-speak" and begin to demystify the common traits of cancer. You won't learn about the particular diagnosed cancer, but about cancer in general, such as:

- The definition of cancer and its origins

- How cancer starts
- What is meant by cancer grading and staging
- What is included in a pathology report

If you are still reeling from a recent cancer diagnosis and would rather do anything other than read an "Intro to Cancer Terminology" chapter, please feel free to skip this chapter and move on to the next one. I felt the same way initially when we first learned of Max's cancer diagnosis but quickly changed my mind when I realized that without a basic understanding of the enemy I would not be able to talk intelligently with her doctors about her condition and treatment.

Remember, *knowledge is power*. With this knowledge of your enemy, you will at least have the ammunition you need to create a fair fight. Go for it!

Defining Cancer

According to the National Cancer Institute (NCI), *cancer* is a term used to define diseases in which abnormal cells divide without control and are able to invade other tissues. Let's look more closely at the components of this definition:

Cancer is a term used to "define diseases." In other words, cancer is not just one disease; it is many diseases. In fact, NCI data identifies more than one hundred different types of cancer.

Cancer cells are "abnormal cells" in the body. What is it that makes these cells abnormal? Unlike normal cells, cancer cells grow and reproduce uncontrollably, *unless they are aggressively treated*. This uncontrolled growth often creates a lump or mass in the body, more commonly known as a tumor.

Cancer cells have the ability to "invade other tissues." They do this in our bodies by traveling through the bloodstream or lymphatic system.

Benign or Malignant Tumors

Not all tumors that appear in the body are cancerous. Some are benign, which means they are composed of normal cells. Benign tumors only cause problems if they increase in size rapidly, interfering with the functioning of a body organ or system. Cancerous or "malignant" tumors are comprised of cancerous cells.

These cells grow at a faster rate than benign tumors, spreading into and destroying surrounding tissues, as well as traveling to other parts of the body. It is the ability cancer cells have to travel throughout the body that makes them such a challenge.

The location where cancer first appears in the body is called the primary cancer. From here, it may spread into nearby body tissues. For example, lung cancer may spread to the spinal cord, as it did in Max's case. Ovarian cancer can spread to the lining of the abdomen (the peritoneum), as it did in Alyson's case. This is called locally advanced cancer. When cancer cells break away from the primary tumor and begin to produce new tumors in other parts of the body, these are called secondary cancers or "metastatic cancer."

Most cancers are named for the organ or type of cell in which they originate. For example, cancer that begins in the breast is called breast cancer; cancer that begins in melanocytes of the skin is called melanoma. NCI places cancer types into the following categories:

- **Carcinoma**—cancer that begins in the skin or in tissues that line or cover internal organs. There are a number of subtypes of carcinoma, including adenocarcinoma, basal cell carcinoma, squamous cell carcinoma, and transitional cell carcinoma.
- **Sarcoma**—cancer that begins in bone, cartilage, fat, muscle, blood vessels, or other connective or supportive tissue.
- **Leukemia**—cancer that starts in blood-forming tissue such as the bone marrow and causes large numbers of abnormal blood cells to be produced and enter the blood.
- **Lymphoma and myeloma**—cancers that begin in the cells of the immune system.
- **Central nervous system cancers**—cancers that begin in the tissues of the brain and spinal cord.

Cancer and Genetics

There is increasing interest on the part of cancer researchers in molecular profiling—testing a tumor for "molecular biomarkers" to help determine the genetic makeup and ideal treatment plan for the tumor(s). Molecular biomarkers are the distinctive fingerprints of gene mutations inside tumor cells that may cause them to be cancerous. To understand exactly how this new research may affect the condition you are dealing with and the treatment, let's take a step back and define the following terms: *genes* and *gene mutations*.

What Are Genes and How Do They Work?

Each cell in our bodies contains genes, coded messages that tell the cell exactly how to behave. Genes make proteins, the building blocks that control a cell's behavior. Each protein has a different function. Some act inside the cell as on and off switches, and it is these proteins that are the focus of much current cancer research.

Sometimes genes malfunction. A malfunction in a gene is called a mutation and is the result of a change in a gene from its natural state or its DNA sequence. Mutations can occur for many reasons, from DNA copying mistakes made during cell division, to exposure to ionizing radiation, to exposure to chemicals called mutagens, or infection by viruses. Cells often destroy themselves if they have a mutation. So most precancerous cells die before they can cause cancer.

Grading, Staging, and Pathology

You may hear your doctor talk about the "grade" of your cancer. This means how developed the cells look under a microscope. Simply put, a low-grade cancer cell looks more like a normal cell and a high-grade cancer cell has an abnormal appearance and is less well developed than a normal cell. Doctors call this distinction between the appearance of cancer cells and normal cells "differentiation." Cells can be well differentiated (low grade or grade 1), moderately differentiated (medium grade or grade 2), or poorly differentiated (high grade or grade 3).

Why Is Grading Important?

Although there are many different ways for cancer cells to behave, grading helps doctors typify their behavior. A low-grade cancer is likely to grow more slowly and be less likely to spread than a high-grade one. Although a doctor cannot be certain exactly how the cancer cells will behave, grade is the best indicator available at the present time.

The doctor dealing with your fight may also mention the stage of the cancer. Staging describes the severity of a person's cancer based on the extent of the original (primary) tumor and whether or not cancer has spread in the body. Doctors use staging as a means of estimating an individual's prognosis. Staging also helps a doctor target the appropriate treatment and identify clinical trials that may be a good match.

The purpose of staging is to help doctors treat their patients. It is useless to compare your cancer "stage" with anyone else's, as everyone's course of treatment and prognosis is different. Staging does not tell the full story, but in the hands of a professional, it is an effective tool.

Staging systems vary according to the type of cancer, but all staging systems report common elements as follows:

- Site of the primary tumor
- Tumor size and number of tumors
- Lymph node involvement (spread of cancer into lymph nodes)
- Cell type and tumor grade
- The presence or absence of metastasis

How Is Stage Determined?

A physical exam is the most common method used to determine the stage of a tumor. Procedures such as X-rays, computed tomography (CT) scans, magnetic resonance imaging (MRI) scans, and positron emission tomography (PET) scans produce pictures of areas inside the body that show the location of the cancer, the size of the tumor, and whether or not the cancer has spread.

Laboratory tests also help stage the tumor. Samples of blood, urine, other fluids, and tissues from the body provide valuable information for doctors to review. Some lab tests are used to measure specific changes in the body, such as increased proteins. These are "tumor markers" and indicate that cancer may be present. These markers may become important later on, as they can be used to detect signs of cancer recurrence.

Tissue specimens are obtained for examination by doing a biopsy, using a needle to withdraw tissue or fluid, or by removing a part of or the entire tumor during surgery. These specimens must be sliced into thin sections before they can be viewed under a microscope. This is known as a histologic (tissue) examination and is usually the best way to tell if cancer is present. The pathologist may also examine cytologic (cell) material. Cytologic material is present in urine, cerebrospinal fluid (the fluid around the brain and spinal cord), sputum (mucus from the lungs), peritoneal (abdominal cavity) fluid, pleural (chest cavity) fluid, cervical/vaginal smears, and in fluid removed during a biopsy.

The Pathologist's Report

After all samples are studied by the pathologist, results are interpreted in a comprehensive pathology report. You may never read your pathology report—or you may decide you want to ask your doctor to see it. In case you choose that course of action, here are some clues for what to look for in your report:

> **Patient information.** Name, birth date, and biopsy date.
> **Gross description.** Color, weight, and size of tissue as seen with the eye.
> **Microscopic description.** How the sample looks under the microscope and compares with normal cells.
> **Diagnosis.** Type of tumor/cancer and grade: how abnormal the cells look under the microscope and how quickly the tumor is likely to grow/spread.
> **Tumor size.** Measured in centimeters.

Tumor margins. There are three possible findings when the biopsy sample is the entire tumor:

- Positive margins mean that cancer cells are found at the edge of the material removed.
- Negative, not involved, clear, or free margins mean that no cancer cells are found at the outer edge.
- Close margins are neither negative nor positive.

Pathologist's signature. Also, the name and address of the laboratory.

The pathologist's job doesn't end here. After identifying the tissue as cancerous, the pathologist may perform additional tests to get further information about the tumor. This is usually information that cannot be determined by looking at the tissue with routine stains under a microscope. Some of these tests help determine where the cancer started and differentiate among different cancer types, such as carcinoma, melanoma, and lymphoma. There are tests that also help diagnose and classify leukemias and lymphomas. The pathology report will also include the results of these additional tests.

The pathology report may also include the results of something called flow cytometry. This is a method of measuring properties of cells in a sample, including the number of cells, percentage of live cells, cell size and shape, and presence of tumor markers on the cell surface. Tumor markers are substances produced by tumor cells or by other cells in the body in response to cancer or certain noncancerous conditions. Flow cytometry can be used in the diagnosis, classification, and management of various types of cancers, including non-Hodgkin's lymphoma and certain types of leukemia.

Finally, the pathology report may include the results of molecular diagnostic and cytogenetic studies. Such studies investigate the presence or absence of malignant cells and genetic or molecular abnormalities.

To Know or Not to Know

Should you ask your doctor about the results of the pathology report? For some, this is a no-brainer. Why not know as much as you can about the condition and diagnosis of the enemy? But not all who are diagnosed with cancer reach this conclusion. Some put all of their faith and trust in the professionals who treat them and have confidence that doctors will tell them all they need to know, when they need to know it.

As for me, I wanted to know for myself. I gobbled up every bit of information I could lay my hands on throughout our long battles with the enemy. I read pathology report after pathology report, as well as all available research on the specific cancer types Max and Alyson were battling.

Would I have done this if I were the patient instead of the patients' "caretaker"? Hard to say, but one thing is certain: whether you put your trust in medical personnel or your own conscientious research, you must face cancer on its own terms. You may as well know what these are.

Final Thoughts: Know Your Enemy

To defeat this enemy, you must get to know the specific type of cancer better than it knows you or your body. Additionally, you must acquire the knowledge to go toe-to-toe with this enemy and the confidence to know that you are making informed decisions at every step in the journey.

Remember

- Becoming familiar with common cancer terms will help to reduce a fear of the unknown.
- The more you know about the enemy, the greater your role can become helping your doctors to select the preferred treatment plan.
- Information is knowledge and knowledge is power.

"Don't take a knife to a gunfight."
—Unknown

Notes

Notes

CHAPTER 4

THE BATTLE PLAN

> *"Planning is bringing the future into the present so that you can do something about it now."*
>
> —Alan Lakein

Patton, starring George C. Scott as the great World War II general, is one of my favorite films. In one famous scene, General George S. Patton stands on a bluff peering through binoculars. He is watching his troops win a decisive victory against the German forces, led by Field Marshal Erwin Rommel (aka the "Desert Fox"). The camera then cuts to a close-up of General Patton looking through his binoculars, as he growls, "Rommel, you magnificent bastard. I read your book." The "book" is Rommel's classic book on military strategy, *Infantry Attacks*. The general knows without a doubt, and so does the audience: he has beaten Rommel at his own game.

Those familiar with military history know the Desert Fox was no ordinary opponent. Up until this point in the war, Field Marshal Rommel had been soundly defeating every Allied general in battle after battle. But General Patton knew better than to engage the Desert Fox without a clear plan that included understanding precisely which moves he would make next. The brilliant U.S. general was well informed and prepared to defeat his enemy.

Failure to Plan Is a Plan to Fail

When battling cancer, it is vitally important that you develop and follow a well-thought-out game plan to determine everything from daily steps to a potential future course of action.

Okay, I admit, it may be a stretch to compare yourself to a great military leader. But think about how valuable good planning has been to you in many aspects of your life. Would you buy a home without first researching the market? Take a family trip without first mapping out the route and a tentative itinerary? In the same vein, does it make sense to engage your enemy without first developing a comprehensive plan of attack?

I have spent most of my professional career leading the design and installation of state-of-the-art computer systems for small- and medium-size businesses. When I found myself face-to-face with this enemy, after the initial shock, I then went into "military mode" and began developing a plan for how I would defeat this enemy. Maybe this sounds a bit cold, but it was the only way I could cope with the overwhelming emotions I felt at the time—by letting the logical side of my brain take over. That turned out to be, in the words of Martha Stewart, "a good thing."

Whether the task is installing a computer system, building a house, or engaging the enemy on the battlefield, the steps for developing a successful plan are similar. Here are some key points for you and your team to think about, as you prepare to draft a customized health battle plan:

- **Keep It Simple.** The KIS formula is the best basis for any plan, as complicated plans tend to cause problems for everyone. The most useful plans are those that are clear, precise, and easy to follow.
- **Keep it brief.** Try to limit your plan to no more than one page for ease of review by you and your team.
- **Keep it basic.** Your plan should list only the basics and be as factual as possible without going into too much detail.

Have supporting notations or documentation available in case it is needed.

Perhaps you are saying to yourself, *"Hold on a minute, Frank, I've never created a plan for anything!"* Have no fear—I have a very simple planning formula to help you easily identify the basic elements included in any successful project plan. Read on!

Writing Your Battle Plan

First, I would like you to get a clean sheet of paper and write across the top these six words: **Who, What, When, Where, Why, How**. These words will prompt you to define the basic elements of your battle plan.

Directly underneath these words, I want you to write the following question: **Will this entry help me to battle this enemy?** This question should be asked and answered in the affirmative for each entry you make in response to each of the six prompt questions. If a question generates a negative or questionable response, do not include it in the plan.

Now, underneath the words and question, I want you to write the first word, **Who.** The "who" element of your plan will allow you to define your primary medical support team. For example, who is/are:

- Your primary doctor(s)
- Oncology team members
- Nationally recognized specialists (for the type of cancer)
- Nationally recognized cancer support organizations
- Family and friends' support team

The beauty of the "who" element is that it allows you to list your key contacts in one place, versus having to shuffle through stacks of papers or business cards every time you require contact information for a key member of your team.

Next, below the "who" question, I want you to write the word **What.** The "what" element of the plan allows you to define the specific area of expertise of each member of your team identified in the prior "who" question. So for example, if you were to list the LIVESTRONG organization in the "who" response, the "what" would be "an organization that is a nationally recognized and leading cancer support and advocacy group." The "what" element helps you clarify your needs and prevents you from duplicating your efforts.

Below the "what," I want you to write the word **When.** The "when" element asks the question, "When should you seek out each individual or organization identified by the 'who' element as a potential resource?" The word *potential* is important here because you are identifying resources you may or may not need. The "when" element allows you to anticipate various scenarios that *may* occur far in the future, including possible alternative treatment options or doctors. This is exactly the kind of strategic thinking that is critical in your battle against this enemy. With this approach, you will be able to adapt quickly on the fly if something is not going as planned. You will not lose precious time trying to make a decision because you will know "when" to use your plan B and already have it in place.

Below the word "when," I want you to write the word **Where.** The "where" element is nothing more than a list of contact information for each individual or organization you have identified as a potential source. Again, you will be thankful that you have this information at your fingertips, should you ever need it.

Below the "where" question, I want you to write the word **Why.** The "why" element requires a little more thought on your part. You will have to think carefully about why you would be contacting or engaging each individual or organization identified in your plan. If you don't have a clear idea of the need for this resource, you may want to remove it for now. Just because a resource isn't listed in your plan, doesn't mean you can't ever use it; you can always resurrect it at some future date. At this point, try to make the plan as streamlined and realistic as possible.

The final word I want you to list on the paper is the word **How.** The "how" element is a reminder of the formal protocol for engaging each individual or organization identified in your plan. Specifically, will you need a referral from a current doctor to see a specialist? What are the requirements of your health plan for each resource listed? Getting this information may seem like a lot of work, but later on, when you are well into your fight, you will be glad to have it at your fingertips.

Congratulations! You have just defined all of the key elements required to create your own personal battle plan. The next challenge is to convert the who, what, when, where, why, and how list into a format that is clear, concise, and easy for you to follow. To assist you in this effort, I have included the plan we developed and used to guide our battle with this formidable enemy.

Short-Term Task Plan—developed and used for our family

Task	Organization	Phone #	Web Address
Identify leading cancer treatment organizations			
	MD Anderson Houston, Texas	877-632-6789	Mdanderson.org
	Mayo Clinic Rochester, Minnesota	507-284-2511	Mayoclinic.org
	Cleveland Clinic Cleveland, Ohio	888-223-2273	Clevelandclinic.org
	Memorial Sloan Kettering New York, New York	800-525-2225	Mskcc.org
	Johns Hopkins Baltimore, Maryland	855-695-4872	Hopkinsmedicine.org
	PinnacleHealth Cancer Center Harrisburg, Pennsylvania	717-657-7500	Pinnaclehealth.org/cancer
Contact family/ friends with cancer treatment experience			
	Relative #1: experience w/ clinical trials @ Sloan Kettering & Johns Hopkins	814 –xxx-xxxx	

KNOW YOUR ENEMY: Taking the Fight to Cancer

	Family friend #1: a leading oncologist specializing in integrative treatment/care	888-xxx-xxxx	
	Family friend #2: a radiologist that will translate "med-speak"	303-xxx-xxxx	
Contact leading cancer support organizations			
	LIVESTRONG: the Lance Armstrong cancer support organization		Livestrong.com
	NavigateCancer Foundation: oncology nurse consultants teamed up w/ LIVESTRONG	919-267-3657	Navigate CancerFoundation.org
	EmergingMed: specialized in clinical trials research, teamed w/ LIVESTRONG	800-620-6167	Emergingmed.com
	Target Now: specialize in molecular profile testing, teamed w/ LIVESTRONG	866-771-8946	Carislifesciences.com
Contact Block Center for integrative treatment program			
(Note: Referred by family friend #1)	A leading integrative cancer treatment center	877-412-5625	Blockmd.com
Make decision on next steps based on findings above			

Final Thoughts: The Battle Plan

General Patton wrote, "A good plan today is better than a perfect plan tomorrow." One of the greatest military strategists of all time, he nevertheless understood that despite best efforts, no one can totally anticipate the future. You create a "working plan" with the information at hand and then adapt your strategy as necessary to meet any changes in the course. If you plan well, you will handle any "surprise attacks" by the enemy with ease.

In our case, the early research and planning efforts became more and more useful, lighting up the way during our darkest times. For me, clarity meant sanity, and sanity meant strength. I sincerely hope that having a battle plan in place does the same for you in your own fight against the enemy.

Remember

- Planning doesn't have to be perfect—just do your best.
- Your plan is a daily "working document," so keep it clear and simple.
- Plan for the future, as well as for the present.

"When a team outgrows individual performance and learns team confidence, excellence becomes a reality."

—Joe Paterno

Notes

Notes

CHAPTER 5

THE SOUL OF BATTLE

"To make our way, we must have firm resolve, persistence, tenacity. We must gear ourselves to work hard all the way. We can never let up."

—Ralph Bunche

On my office wall hangs a poster of my favorite Boston Celtics player: Larry Bird or Larry Legend to the Celtics faithful. The poster depicts Bird shooting a jump shot over the outstretched arm of some faceless and nameless defender. The look in Larry's eyes tells the story of why the poster reads *Larry Bird DETERMINATION* and includes the following definition of **determination**: "1. The quality of being firm in purpose or action; resoluteness. 2. To commit oneself to a goal or action."

The point of this story and the chapter introductory quote is to emphasize that there are things in this battle that you can control and other things that are beyond your control. Your ability to focus your energy and efforts on the things you can control—your attitude, your effort, your determination, your commitment—will go a long way toward helping you to defeat this enemy.

I have included inspirational messages from three well-known coaches to illustrate further the importance of these core attributes.

As you read, try to picture yourself sitting in a locker room, with the other members of your cancer-fighting team, listening to each coach deliver their impassioned message about how these attributes can help you in both sports and life.

"Don't Give Up…Don't Ever Give Up." —Jim Valvano

I was flipping through the channels one night in early March of 1993 and happened to come across a special on ESPN called the ESPY Awards. The ESPY (Excellence in Sports Performance Yearly) Award is presented to recognize team and individual athletic achievement during a given year. What I didn't realize at the time was that this was the first ever ESPY Awards and that what I was about to hear would be remembered as one of the most inspirational speeches ever.

James Thomas Anthony "Jim" Valvano, nicknamed Jimmy V, the legendary American NCAA men's college-basketball coach and broadcaster, was being presented with the inaugural Arthur Ashe Courage and Humanitarian Award. While accepting the award, he announced the creation of The V Foundation for Cancer Research, an organization dedicated to finding a cure for cancer. The foundation's motto would be "Don't Give Up…Don't Ever Give Up."

Jimmy V closed his moving speech with these words: "Cancer can take away all of my physical abilities. It cannot touch my mind, it cannot touch my heart, and it cannot touch my soul. And those three things are going to carry on forever. I thank you and God bless you all." At the end of the speech, he was escorted from the stage to a standing ovation. There was not a dry eye in the house.

I encourage you to go to your computer and do an Internet search for "Jim Valvano's 1993 ESPN ESPY Awards speech," and then watch it. Have plenty of tissues on hand because Jimmy V is going to make you both laugh and cry. Secondly, if the spirit moves you, go to The V Foundation for Cancer Research website at www.JimmyV.org and make a donation to an excellent organization and cause.

It helps to remember Jimmy V's words as you begin your battle against the enemy. Cancer may ravage your body, but it cannot touch your heart or your soul. During our long battle, these are the words I lived by. However, none of this is to say battling cancer is easy. It is true that cancer cannot touch your heart or your soul, but you will need both to defeat it.

"...they are who we thought they were! And we let 'em off the hook!" —Dennis Green

Coach Dennis Green provided us with an inspiring moment on the importance of firm resolve, persistence, and perseverance after a stinging loss on Monday Night Football in 2006. The Chicago Bears had just defeated the Arizona Cardinals. The Cardinals, coached by Dennis Green, had given up a twenty-point lead in less than twenty minutes of play. In responding to a series of postgame media questions about the loss, the usually congenial Green erupted:

> *"The Bears are who we thought they were! That's why we took the damn field! Now if you want to crown them, then crown their @#$ but they are who we thought they were! And we let 'em off the hook!"*

Coach Green's outburst was a surprise, due to his usually calm public demeanor; however, it was clear he had something important to say, something that is still frequently used in NFL media coverage when one team recognizes the obvious flaws in an opponent but fails to capitalize on this knowledge.

To me, his words capture the raw frustration, and disappointment, from not seeing his players put their minds, hearts, and souls into winning. What I hear behind Coach Green's words are the words he may have thought, but didn't say:

> *"We, as a coaching staff and players, poured our hearts and souls into game-planning against the Chicago Bears. We then successfully executed our game plan for three quarters. And yet, when it came time to put the game away, we were not able to finish the task, and this attitude of self-defeat allowed our opponent to come back and beat us."*

You see, Coach Green's team had known the enemy ("The Bears are who we thought they were"), and they had known themselves ("That's why we took the damn field"), yet they had still lost the game. What they lacked was persistence—the persistence of heart and soul that brings spirit to the fight and a refusal to give up until the very end.

"You play to win the game." —Herman Edwards, Jr.

At a 2002 press conference, former NFL player, and then head coach of the New York Jets, Herman Edwards, Jr. gave us insight into the competitive nature of the NFL and the importance of hard work. Coach Edwards was responding to a question about the team's work ethic and commitment to winning. Some found his response that contained the now-famous "you play to win the game" quote humorous. However, as I watched the clip in its entirety (at least ten times!), I began to understand the wisdom in his words and why they might be valuable for those fighting this enemy. Here is his statement in its entirety:

> *"You don't get to quit. It's not an option…that ain't even an option…This is what the greatest thing about sports is, you play to win the game… You play to win, and I don't care if you don't have any wins, you go play to win. When you start telling me it doesn't matter, then retire. Get out, because it matters. This whole conversation bothers me, big time. It really does. Because the one thing I know, I don't quit. That will not happen. That will not happen."*

In Coach Edwards' statement, I hear the competitive juices flowing of an ex-NFL player that would love nothing more than the opportunity to put on the uniform just one more time and compete. The life lesson that I believe Coach Edwards, Coach Green, or any other great coach will tell you regarding competing is that when you get your opponent down and on the ropes, you must finish them off. You cannot let 'em off the hook or quit before the task is completed.

The same is true when battling your personal enemy—cancer. If you begin to see positive results from your treatment program, most coaches would tell you that rather than viewing this as an opportunity to coast or take a time-out, you should instead view it as an opening to dial up the intensity level. In football-coach-speak, they would probably say something like this:

> *"You need to put on your big-boy shoulder pads, buckle up your chin strap, and get back in the game and take it to the opponent over and over again, until we have imposed our will on them."*

Final Thoughts: The Soul of Battle

I've attempted to lighten up what is a serious topic through the use of famous sports figures and their respective quotes. The bottom line: you are fighting cancer in the real-world arena called life. The stakes are high, and there are very few instances, in this game, where you will get a second chance once you've heard the sound of the starter's gun. Persistence, perseverance, and a dogged determination may be the best skills you have in your arsenal against cancer. All you can do is your best, put your heart and soul into it, and don't give up—don't *ever* give up!

Remember

- Give one hundred percent to the battle.
- Quitting is not an option.
- No one ever said it was going to be easy.

"Whether you think you can or think you can't, either way you are right."

—Henry Ford

I had an IBM colleague and friend from the Windy City who was going through a difficult stretch at one point in her life. I was really feeling for her and wrote the following little pick-me-up piece to lift her spirits. I think the message of persistence and perseverance fits nicely with the points of emphasis in this chapter and hope that it helps others facing difficult times.

Untitled

When times get tough, as they often do,
Plant your feet firmly, you're going to make it through.
Dig down deep inside, and don't be afraid to cry.
But whatever you do, don't ever ask why.
Remember what got you this far, you made it on your own.
But also remember family and friends are here,
to make sure you're not fighting alone.
Today the chips seem down, but tomorrow's a new day.
And you know what you have to look forward
to, everything finally going your way!

Notes

Notes

CHAPTER 6

TIMING IS EVERYTHING

"Time is the wisest counselor of all."
—Pericles

Like most business consultants, I have learned that when it comes to capturing the market, timing is everything. If I enter the market with a new service before the public is ready, I am likely to fall flat on my face. If I enter the market too late, I risk losing out to another service provider. This principle of the right timing is also an important military strategy and one of the most important lessons in *The Art of War*. Sun Tzu called this understanding—of when to hold back and when to take action—"tien."

Time and Timing

You've heard the expression "lie in wait." What this means, according to my online free dictionary, is to "stay hidden, ready to attack" or to "delay doing something until the best time for it." Good timing is important in your battle against the enemy. Timing refers to anticipating change and taking appropriate action when it's most needed. Is it a good time to switch to a new treatment? Would a different doctor be to your advantage? You have everything at your disposal that you need to make the right choice at the right time. Use your battle plan as a safety net.

Trust your "balanced mind" and move forward without hesitation when the time feels right.

Time, as it relates to your battle against cancer, also refers to the endless amount of time spent in doctors' offices, hospitals, or other medical facilities. If you're not spending your time attending rounds of appointments, then you are spending hours scheduling them or traveling from one to the next. Or you're spending time waiting—for the next treatment, doctor's appointment, test result, etc. As anyone who has battled this enemy knows, there is a significant amount of "downtime" in treatment. What you do with this downtime is just as significant a strategy as knowing when to choose a new doctor or treatment center.

Sometimes, time can be your enemy. But when it comes to cancer treatment, you can make time your friend. Instead of allowing unproductive blocks of time in your schedule to introduce fear of the unknown, uncertainty, and anxiety, use these blocks of time as windows of opportunity. Then, like every good general, you will thwart the enemy's intentions, using downtime to gain the advantage.

Here are some ideas for you and your family that I hope will help you to use time to your advantage. Remember to spend as much time in the active mode as possible to defend your position against the enemy.

Know your time frame. Waiting for the results of a biopsy or some other test can be especially challenging. As anyone who has been through it knows, it can be nerve-racking waiting for the news and hard not to let fear and an active imagination get the better of you. One way to relieve this stress is always to ask the doctor when you can expect to receive test results. Having a specific date and time frame allows you to reduce some of the anxiety that may occur when the wait is longer than you expected.

Keep one step ahead. Knowing your enemy means anticipating his next move. Make sure you are aware of the next steps in your health process. Always have a list of questions for each doctor based upon the next steps in the process. For example, you might want to know, based upon test results, what the options are going forward and the associated next steps for each option. The more that you know regarding the specific medical condition, treatment program, and current health status, the better—not just for you, but also for the medical team, including doctors, family members, and friends.

Use time to your advantage. I encourage you to think of blocks of downtime as your own special "time-outs." Consider each waiting period as a mini mental-health break and look forward to the opportunity to recharge your battery—you will need it! Escape to a book, magazine, movie, or if you're able enough, enjoy dinner out. Catch up on your e-mails or balance your checkbook. Keep a journal of your activities and progress. Send a card or letter to a friend you haven't seen or talked to in quite a while. Activities such as these provide an ideal outlet and distraction from the daily battle you're engaged in.

During Alyson's battle with cancer, I learned to turn our blocks of downtime into productive and even enjoyable experiences. I wrote the majority of the first draft of this book while we were flying back and forth to the Block Center in Chicago, where Alyson had her specialized treatment. I would take out a pen and scratch paper anytime the spirit moved me—in airports, on flights, in hotels, while Alyson was receiving chemotherapy. I also relied heavily on working out and spent a lot of time doing P90X and walking/jogging outside to clear my mind. I needed an outlet to reduce the stress, tension, and pressure; fortunately, I found it.

Make downtime "real time." As the old football saying goes, "Focus on one play at a time and just do your job." Don't worry about the previous play—that is in the past—or the next play. This coaching philosophy recognizes that the only thing players can control is how well they perform their respective assignment on the current play called. If all eleven players execute their individual assignment to a high degree, then the outcome should, more often than not, be a successful play. This is good advice for the entire health journey. Focus your energy on the task at hand and make your decisions based upon the here and now, versus the future, and what may or may not happen. Try to live by the mantra of one day or one play at a time.

Final Thoughts: Timing Is Everything

With a cancer diagnosis, you may feel that time is suddenly more precious and that you don't want to waste a minute. You can't wait for all to be well again to get on with your life, yet you are forced to wait, and wait, through the long process of treatment. For most people, this wait is grueling—I know it was for us. To cope, we found a way to make these times less stressful, and in the end, the minutes and hours spent together waiting became a source of joy and happiness. I encourage you to do the same.

Remember

- Right timing is important in any battle. Trust your instincts.
- Take it one day at a time; don't look back or rush forward.
- Use downtime to recharge your battery.

"All of life is peaks and valleys. Don't let the peaks get too high and the valleys too low."

—John Wooden

Notes

Notes

CHAPTER 7

GATHERING INTEL

"Just the facts, ma'am."
—Sergeant Joe Friday, from the TV show *Dragnet*

In the days of the Civil War, generals received military intelligence in a variety of ways. Spies and scouts played vital roles, reporting directly to field commanders and relaying important details on troop movements and strengths. We still have our spies; but these days, military leaders rely on an increasingly sophisticated network of military intelligence to ferret out an opponent's plans of attack. We are, of course, in the information age, and there is a deluge of information available—some of it more reliable than others. That is why it is necessary to have trusted sources—those that can be counted on during these critical times.

In your battle against the enemy, you will likely have no shortage of information available to you. This information will come from a variety of sources: your physicians and other medical personnel, your friends and family, and of course, the Internet. One of your greatest challenges will be to determine which of these sources is likely to provide you with the best information and which you can trust.

The Trusted Advisor

In his classic book *The Trusted Advisor*, David Meister writes of the necessity for an individual in business to earn the trust of his clients. He describes "the trusted advisor" as "the person the client turns to when an issue first arises, often in times of great urgency: a crisis, a change, a triumph, or a defeat."

As I mentioned before, I became aware, very early on in this battle, that we would need to create our own list of "trusted advisors"—a team of medical professionals that would support us in our effort to battle the enemy. These would be individuals we could call on with confidence, no matter what happened, through good times and bad. I realized how fortunate we were even to have this option. It hadn't been all that long ago when a diagnosis of cancer meant that nothing could be done. Now we would have our very own team in place to guide us through this warzone.

Perhaps you have already started to assemble your own team of trusted advisors. As you move along in this battle, I predict you will rely more and more on the team you have created to give you good advice, make you aware of promising new treatments, and reassure you in challenging times.

Your trusted advisors are clearly your most valued information resource in the days ahead, especially regarding your specific form of cancer and its treatment.

But these days, it's impossible not to want to use the Internet as a research tool. It's just too tempting to turn on the computer and surf away! All I have to say on this subject is "go for it," but make sure you are fully aware of the risks attached.

Using the Internet for Medical Research

The strength and limitation of the Internet are two sides of the same coin: the vastness of available content and the pollution of much of that content. To use the Internet as an effective medical research tool, you will have to separate the wheat from the chaff—to harness the Internet's great power but still manage to steer clear of unreliable sources and content.

As long as you are aware of the pitfalls, the Internet can be a valuable asset in your battle against the enemy. I encourage you to use the Internet to:

- accelerate your understanding of basic or introductory cancer terminology;
- become familiar with new medical terminology that will help you understand tests, procedures, chemo drugs, or other information presented to you;
- identify support organizations and their services available to you; and
- identify the medical hospitals and professionals that specialize in your cancer treatment.

I'm sure you have experienced logging on to the Internet with a specific purpose in mind, only to find yourself, several hours later, shopping for clothes or reading someone's blog. How can you use the Internet as a helpful research tool and avoid getting sidetracked in this way? To use the Internet for medical research, you must be purposeful and single-minded. I found it helpful to use a three-prong formula that has worked for me throughout my professional career. I believe anyone can adopt this same approach and find success.

Be specific. Start your Internet research with a predefined purpose, e.g., investigating the treatment options for a specific type of cancer. If you make your searches as specific as possible, then you will yield better results.

Be finite. Have a "starting point" and "end point" to each search: begin with a limited number of broad search queries (starting point) until you are able to identify the website(s) that can answer your questions. When you find the answers or information you are seeking, immediately document your findings (end point).

Be minimal. Keep the topics being researched within the same subject matter and limit their number to three. This technique allows you to reduce or at least minimize the opportunities for straying into the Internet "unknown" when you are performing your search queries.

One last thought: Although it may be tempting to look up statistics relating to the prognosis of the particular type of cancer you are fighting, I hope I can dissuade you from this activity. When it comes to cancer, there is no "one size fits all." Statistics found on the Internet tend to be "mass averages" bearing little relationship to your unique situation. Additionally, I am of the belief that any findings or statistics that may introduce anxiety or fear to an already tense situation should be avoided at all costs.

Consider the Alternatives

There is still no "magic bullet" to eradicate cancer, yet in laboratories all over the world, recent research—especially in the area of gene targeting—shows that huge progress is being made. What is clear is that (1) with every passing day, new options for treatment present themselves for cancer and of every type and (2) not all of the treatment options available to you will come under the heading of "traditional" medicine. If you want to consider alternative approaches, you may have to go "outside the lines" to find out what is available in your case, but perhaps you will feel it is worth the effort.

During my two battles with the enemy, I did extensive treatment research to make sure we knew all options available for both my mother and my wife. While I tended to be more in the traditionalist camp, and mainly considered these types of alternatives, I did identify and we considered a wide range of treatment options.

The following charts show (1) the leading national organizations on the frontlines in this battle against cancer and (2) the many treatment options available within each organization.

Cancer Research and Treatment Organizations Identified During Our Battles

Organization	Location	Phone #	Web Address
MD Anderson	Houston, Texas	877-632-6789	Mdanderson.org
Mayo Clinic	Rochester, Minnesota	507-284-2511	Mayoclinic.org
Cleveland Clinic	Cleveland, Ohio	888-223-2273	Clevelandclinic.org
Memorial Sloan-Kettering	New York, New York	800-525-2225	Mskcc.org
Johns Hopkins Hospital	Baltimore, Maryland	855-695-4872	Hopkinsmedicine.org
PinnacleHealth Cancer Center	Harrisburg, Pennsylvania	717-657-7500	Pinnaclehealth.org/cancer
Harbin Clinic	Rome, Georgia	888-427-2461	Harbinclinic.com
The Block Center	Skokie, Illinois	877-412-5625	Blockmd.com

Cancer Patient Advocate and Support Organizations

Support/Organization	Location	Phone #	Web Address
Clearinghouse: LIVESTRONG Foundation	Austin, Texas	877-236-8820	Livestrong.org
Nurse Support Services: NavigateCancer	Apex, North Carolina	866-391-1121	Navigatecancerfoundation.org
Clinical Trials Clearinghouse: EmergingMed	New York, New York	800-620-6167	Emergingmed.com
Molecular Profile Testing: Caris Life Sciences	Phoenix, Arizona	866-771-8946	Carislifesciences.com

Pennsylvania Cyberknife Robotic Radiosurgery Center

Organization	Location	Phone #	Web Address
PinnacleHealth Cancer Center	Harrisburg, Pennsylvania	717-657-7500	Pinnaclehealth.org/cancer

Cancer Research Foundation

Organization	Location	Phone #	Web Address
The V Foundation for Cancer Research	Cary, North Carolina	919-380-9505	Jimmyv.org

In considering the alternatives, don't reject ideas just because they sound "weird." Paul McCartney was once quoted as saying, *"I used to think anyone doing anything weird was weird. I suddenly realized that anyone doing anything weird wasn't weird at all, and it was the people saying they were weird that were weird."*

This is your battle, your treatment. I advise you not to worry about being considered "weird." Above all else, keep an open mind. Don't hesitate to research treatment options that may be available to complement the more traditional approaches.

Final Thoughts: Gathering Intel

I hope you realize that when it comes to seeking out the information you need to fight this enemy, there is no intelligence greater than your own. Your resolve to defeat this enemy results from your own diligent efforts as well as from the support of the trusted advisors you assemble.

Remember

- Build a team of trusted advisors you can go to with confidence.
- Harness the power of the Internet, but avoid its pitfalls.
- Consider all resources available—traditional and nontraditional.

"If everyone is thinking alike, then somebody isn't thinking."

—George S. Patton

Notes

Notes

CHAPTER 8

THE POWER OF FAITH

> *"Faith is taking the first step even when you don't see the whole staircase."*
>
> —Martin Luther King, Jr.

I believe it's important for any individual battling cancer, or any major health challenge, to have a spiritual component to his or her battle plan. Faith does not place the value of one religion over another; in fact, it need not mean organized religion of any kind. I'm using the word *faith* in the context of having a spiritual foundation based on a belief in a greater being and purpose in life.

Abraham Lincoln was private about his religious beliefs—yet he acknowledged on several occasions the presence and importance of faith in battle. In one such statement, made to General Dan Sickles, while referring to the Battle of Gettysburg, Lincoln said the following:

> *"Well, I will tell you how it was. In the pinch of the campaign up there (at Gettysburg) when everybody seemed panic stricken and nobody could tell what was going to happen, oppressed by the gravity of our affairs, I went to my room one day and locked the*

door and got down on my knees before Almighty God and prayed to Him mightily for victory at Gettysburg…And after that, I don't know how it was, and I cannot explain it, but soon a sweet comfort crept into my soul." (July 5, 1863)

During my family's battles with the enemy, we relied upon our faith to help get us through each day. Were there times when we were less upbeat and optimistic about the events of the day? Of course. We had our share of difficult moments, but our faith always provided us with a floor to rebound from and enabled us to reset our emotions for the next day, and the next.

On the flip side, our faith also lightened our spirits and helped us to appreciate and to savor each victory, regardless of the experience—a good therapy session, receiving positive treatment results, or simply a general improvement in Max's or Alyson's health. If there was something positive to celebrate, then celebrate we did!

Max drew special comfort from the words of the prayers she loved. When Alyson was first diagnosed, she asked me for Max's Bible. She kept it by her bedside throughout her treatment and read it on a regular basis. We never discussed it, but I believe she took comfort from Max's strength, and having her Bible seemed to give Alyson a spiritual confidence to face whatever might come.

Lastly, faith can help you to both recognize the goodness in others and, equally as important, the benefit you will receive from helping your loved ones in need. Directing your thoughts and efforts toward helping others can oftentimes be the best and least expensive self-healing remedy. We felt truly blessed by the care and compassion others demonstrated toward my mother and my wife during their time of need.

Final Thoughts: The Power of Faith

Whether you are a believer in a specific religion or you have an individual spiritual guide, your type of faith can bring you some peace. The idea is not to use faith as a crutch. Once you have given it all you have got and have put every ounce of your energy into the fight, you gain peace by putting whatever is to happen in the hands of a spiritual force greater than your own.

Remember

- Faith comes in many forms.
- We all find faith in our own time and in our own way.
- Faith may help give you a positive attitude that allows you to keep going.

"God grant me the serenity to accept the things I cannot change; courage to change the things I can; and wisdom to know the difference."

—Theologian Reinhold Niebuhr

Notes

Notes

CHAPTER 9

WINNING IS A MINDSET

*"Push yourself again and again.
Don't give an inch until the final buzzer sounds."*

—Larry Bird

There is a verse in the intro to Aerosmith's "Dream On"— *"You got to lose to know how to win."* That is one of my favorite lines in a song. For me, this phrase captures my life lessons learned, as well as what I took away from both encounters with this enemy. I've found that very few successes in life, at least for me, have come without hard work, sacrifice, overcoming adversity, and in most cases rebounding from a loss or setback. In terms of battling this enemy, I believe that *you've got to lose* or give up the sense of being in control or controlling the treatment, time frame, or outcome *to ultimately know how* to prepare yourself *to win* your battle against this enemy.

What Exactly Does It Mean <u>To Win</u>?

Seldom does the topic of winning come up without mention of the famous quote attributed to the legendary head coach of the Green

Bay Packers, Vince Lombardi: *"Winning isn't everything; it's the only thing."* And yet, according to Coach Lombardi himself, this quote may be one of the most misinterpreted and misunderstood quotes of the modern era.

In the documentary titled *Lombardi*, Jerry Izenberg, a sportswriter from Lombardi's native New Jersey, recounts a conversation he had with Coach Lombardi that sheds light on the belief system of the coach. "(Lombardi) told me once, 'I wish to hell I'd never said, "Winning isn't everything…it's the only thing."' I (Mr. Izenberg) then said, 'Don't you believe it?' He said, 'What I believe is, if you go out on a football field, or any endeavor in life, and you leave every fiber of what you have on the field, then you've won.'"

To me, this battle we've been talking about isn't "won" in the traditional sense. I believe, as Coach Lombardi, that *to win* means being a true warrior in your mindset and approach to battling this enemy, as I have described throughout this book. It means having the physical and mental toughness to take this enemy head-on, with every fiber of your being, each and every day. And it means enlisting the support of close family and friends ("gathering your troops") and relying on your faith to help you battle this enemy. Additionally, it means leaving nothing on the table in terms of the specialists you engage and treatment you pursue. Another highly successful football coach, Paul "Bear" Bryant, put it this way: *"If you believe in yourself and have dedication and pride—and never quit, you'll be a winner. The price of victory is high but so are the rewards."* In the end, if you are able to adopt these basic principles, you are certain to "win" the battle against this enemy.

Final Thoughts: Winning Is a Mindset

If you were to ask me what is the one thing I should take away from this chapter or the book, I would have to say it is the understanding that in cancer, as in life, there are many factors beyond your control—stage, type, detection, genetic composition, environment, diet, fate, etc.—and ultimately all of these X factors will play a role in determining the outcome of your battle. Do all that you can—*all that you must*—to fight this enemy. But when the going gets tough, as The Serenity Prayer says, know that there are some things you can control and some that you can't. That is the secret to standing tall against the enemy. That is how, ultimately, you "win."

Remember

- Take the fight to this enemy each and every day.
- Seek the best specialists and treatments for your specific type of cancer.
- Accept the fact that some health issues may fall beyond your control.

"The difference between ordinary and extraordinary is that little extra."

—James William "Jimmy" Johnson (American Football Coach)

It seems fitting to close this chapter with the poem "The Guy in the Glass," about what it really means to be a winner. Legend has it that the poem was first discovered scrawled on the wall of a death-row prison cell in San Quentin. In reality, the poem was written by Dale Wimbrow and first published in 1934. I learned of it during a documentary on Bill Parcells, two-time Super Bowl–winning coach for the New York Giants. Coach Parcells had read the poem to his team prior to announcing his retirement.

For me, this poem captures the true spirit of my mother, my wife, and all modern-day cancer-fighting warriors. I hope that it moves you as much as it did me.

The Guy in the Glass

When you get what you want in your struggle for pelf,
And the world makes you King for a day,
Then go to the mirror and look at yourself,
And see what that guy has to say.
For it isn't your Father, or Mother, or Wife,
Who judgement upon you must pass.
The feller whose verdict counts most in your life
Is the guy staring back from the glass.
He's the feller to please, never mind all the rest,
For he's with you clear up to the end,
And you've passed your most dangerous, difficult test
If the guy in the glass is your friend.
You may be like Jack Horner and "chisel" a plum,
And think you're a wonderful guy,
But the man in the glass says you're only a bum
If you can't look him straight in the eye.
You can fool the whole world down the pathway of years,
And get pats on the back as you pass,
But your final reward will be heartaches and tears
If you've cheated the guy in the glass.

Notes

Notes

CHAPTER 10

I'M STILL STANDING

"It's not whether you get knocked down; it's whether you get back up."
—Vince Lombardi

If you or a loved one recently received a cancer diagnosis, your world has literally been turned upside down overnight. The only difference between you and me might be that I was faced with this same experience not once but twice, within a seven-month period. Did these personal hardships knock me on my tail? You bet they did—the first time. But upon receiving the bad news for the second time, I told myself, *"Okay, Frank, you know the drill,"* and I DID. I was ready to take the fight to cancer.

As Coach Vince Lombardi said in the famous quote stated above, *"It's not whether you get knocked down; it's whether you get back up,"* and guess what? *I'm still standing!* I've been shocked, kicked, and punched in the gut; but the enemy hasn't defeated me. Not only have I stood my ground, but also I've morphed into a new, confident individual, able to withstand just about anything the enemy can throw at me, and then some.

On top of that, my views on life and my priorities have completely evolved. You might say I now have my own set of "Post-Cancer Guiding Principles":

1. Focus on the present.
2. Make time for people who make time for you.
3. Live for today. *Carpe diem.*
4. Always act decisively and with conviction.

Rule #1: Focus on the present.

There is a scene from the movie *The Gumball Rally* that drives, pardon the pun, this point home. The rally participants are gathered in a New York City garage prior to the start of the race when the camera cuts to the cockpit of a bright red Ferrari Daytona convertible. The Ferrari driver, a "top-gun" Italian racer, looks at his copilot and, as he rips the rearview mirror off the windshield, says the first rule of Italian driving is "Whatsa behind me is not important."

Now, don't get me wrong: There is certainly value in learning from previous mistakes. In fact, *I believe you can never really move forward in your life until you come to terms with your past.* But then, once you do, it's equally important to move on and *live again*. No matter what the consequence of your battle with the enemy, you have to walk off the battlefield, pick up the reins of your life, and focus on what's happening right now.

Rule #2: Make time for people who make time for you.

I'm blessed with having the greatest collection of friends (including Simon the Cat), some going back as far as elementary school to post college. The common trait among my friends, beyond the obvious—they are great people, is that they are "givers" versus "takers." Givers are individuals that influence your life in a positive manner. They are unselfish with their time and have a genuine concern and empathy for anyone confronted with a major life challenge.

During my two battles with the enemy, my friends just "knew" when I needed reinforcements, and time and again, one or several of the guys would show up without a phone call or text from me. This special bond and brotherhood motivated me to write the poem "The Chosen Few," mentioned in chapter 1.

I've always been good about staying in touch with and helping my friends. But I can tell you that post-cancer, when I have an opportunity to get together with a friend(s) or to help a friend in need, I don't wait to be asked—I take the initiative and do it! I would do anything for this group of special guys, and I would encourage you to do the same for the special individuals in your life.

Rule #3: Live for today. *Carpe diem*.

In your battle against the enemy, I encourage you to spend a lot of time thinking, planning, and researching. But once the battle is over, you need to start *doing* again. Stop looking for reasons not to do things, but rather seek justification and support for why you should act. It's time! When you are able to move on from the past, you need to make your way again among the living. Get out and enjoy your life.

Let me give you a couple of examples of how this post-cancer change in philosophy has positively impacted my life. Prior to this experience, the following items would have been found on my "wish list." Now they can be found on my "recent accomplishments list." I want to:

- ✓ complete the writing of this book and get it published,
- ✓ create more entertainment space in the house for friends and family,
- ✓ sell my limited-use, award-winning 1964 Corvette,
- ✓ pursue the formal project management certification,
- ✓ go to NASCAR's "Mecca" Talladega to see a race, and
- ✓ take guitar lessons—need to find a good teacher.

Rule #4: Always act decisively and with conviction.

My home office, where I'm currently drafting this chapter, has an IBM THINK sign, from my days at IBM, proudly displayed on top of the bookcase. The IBM THINK sign became a one-word motivational slogan for the company after Thomas J. Watson reported at a sales conference, *"Thought has been the father of every advance since time began. 'I didn't think' has cost the world millions of dollars."* Then, he took out a blue crayon, and wrote the word "THINK." Up until our two battles with cancer, that word T-H-I-N-K had been my mantra. Now, I would have to add the word A-C-T. It was my ability to A-C-T during those stressful days that made me feel I was truly on top of my game and "in the zone." My high level of concentration allowed me not only to research, plan, and THINK, but also to ACT quickly and confidently. As a result, I was able to hold my own with the best and brightest minds in the medical profession.

Post-cancer, this newfound confidence continues. I'm no longer just going through the motions of life or coasting. I'm actively living my life, doing what I want to do, when I want, with whomever I want. Cancer has given me the confidence not just to THINK but also to ACT.

Final Thoughts: I'm Still Standing

The battle you face is like no other and isn't "won" or "lost" in conventional ways. Knowing this at the outset is the secret to "defeating this enemy" and will keep you from losing your way when times are tough.

As you move on, you may want to keep the immortal words of the great hockey-player-turned-coach Wayne Gretzky in mind: *"A good hockey player plays where the puck is. A great hockey player plays where the puck is going to be."*

Look forward, and enjoy the journey.

Remember

- To really move forward in life, one must first come to terms with the past.
- Make time for special friends and family members.
- Live for today!

"Today, you have 100% of your life left."

—Tom Landry

Notes

Notes

EPILOGUE

LAST WORDS

"Precious and few are the moments we two can share."
—Lyrics to the song "Precious and Few" (recorded by Climax)

One of my earliest memories of hearing the word *cancer* comes from the 1971 made-for-TV movie *Brian's Song*. This movie is the story of the special friendship between Gale Sayers, Pro Football Hall of Fame running back for the Chicago Bears, and his fellow teammate, roommate, and running back, Brian Piccolo.

The movie depicts two highly competitive men, Gale Sayers (played by Billy Dee Williams) and Brian Piccolo (played by James Caan), initially competing for the same starting tailback spot on the Chicago Bears roster. When Gale injures his knee, Brian, in a special act of kindness and compassion, takes a weight machine to Gale's house to aid his rehab effort. Gale makes a full recovery, and for a short time, both men share the backfield for the Bears, as the starting tailback and fullback.

Their bond grows stronger when Brian is hospitalized due to weight loss, and then receives word of a cancer diagnosis. In an emotional locker-room speech, Gale makes teammates aware of

Brian's serious health condition and later takes a game ball to Brian in the hospital.

In one of the final scenes, Gale tells the attendees of the George S. Halas Most Courageous Player Award ceremony that they have selected the wrong person for the award and dedicates his speech to honoring his teammate and friend. He closes a heartfelt speech with the following words, *"I love Brian Piccolo, and I'd like all of you to love him, too. Tonight, when you hit your knees to pray, please ask God to love him, too."*

The movie ends showing a flashback of Brian Piccolo and Gale Sayers running through the park while a narrator says that Brian died at age twenty-six and is remembered as he lived, rather than how he died.

Brian's Song is one of the few tearjerker movies that I would watch every time it was on TV. Why was I so drawn to this movie? Because, to me, it captures the selfless nature and compassionate acts of two special men that put friendship and the needs of a fellow teammate above personal gain or individual accolades.

Fast-forward forty-plus years and now it was my family that was confronted with fighting this enemy not once but twice in less than twelve months. This forced us, out of necessity, to learn more than we ever wanted to know about this enemy. And then I experienced an "aha" moment in my living room, during my wife's battle, and the idea for what would eventually become this book first entered my mind. In that instance, I was given the title and subtitle for the book—***Know Your Enemy: Taking the Fight to Cancer***—along with ideas for chapter titles.

I never intended to write a book, let alone a cancer book. And yet each time I sat down to write it was as if the words were flowing through me and I was merely the vehicle or tool to capture this information. When people ask, "What made you think you could write a book about cancer?" I tell them that I didn't write this book; it was written through me.

As the book began to take shape, I had three goals: (1) to complete the project, if nothing else for my own sense of accomplishment, (2) to share my cancer-fighting experiences with other first-time cancer patients (family members and caregivers) to help them jumpstart their process of getting to *know the enemy—cancer*, and (3) to ensure that each chapter provided readers with a message of inspiration and hope, as the movie *Brian's Song* did for me. I wanted to leave readers with a sense of optimism as they embarked on their respective journey, without sugarcoating the realities of my mother's and my wife's battles with this enemy.

In the introduction, I talked about how this enemy attacked Max and Alyson and my reaction to hearing "The Word"—CANCER—for the first time. I have purposely waited until this point in the book to share the outcome of these battles.

My mother, Max, was rushed to the hospital Labor Day, Monday, 2011. She had to have emergency spinal surgery to remove the part of the tumor that was pressing against the spine. Following the surgery, Max undertook an intensive twelve-week, seven-days-a-week physical and occupational therapy program. She progressed from being unable to use her legs to beginning to walk with limited assistance from her therapist. Three weeks after her surgery, Max also began receiving daily radiation treatments (39) combined with weekly chemo treatments (7). She never missed a treatment and her final CT scan showed a significant shrinkage in the tumor.

Our family had a very special Thanksgiving holiday, and we were looking forward to Max being released from the hospital just in time for Christmas. In early December, however, she began to have breathing problems. The doctors initially thought Max had a bad case of pneumonia. We later learned that she had contracted a very rare lung condition (interstitial lung disease) believed to be the result of trauma to the lungs.

Max battled this enemy with a warriorlike mental, physical, and emotional toughness; and as the subtitle of this book states, she took the fight to cancer! While her earthly being is no longer with us, Max passed on Saturday, December 17, 2011, her spirit lives on in my heart and mind.

My wife, Alyson, was referred to a cancer specialist at the Milton S. Hershey Medical Center. Upon receiving the news from the doctor that the growth was squamous cell carcinoma, he recommended a radical hysterectomy, followed by an aggressive chemo treatment plan. After three cycles with the first chemo cocktail, the CT scan results showed additional "new" growths. The same protocol was followed with a second chemo cocktail. The test results again showed no impact on the disease.

At this point, we felt that it was time for a major change. I reached out to our good friend Dr. Mumber and he referred Alyson to the Block Center in Illinois, one of the world's leading cancer treatment facilities—specializing in individualized programs designed to give patients the best opportunity to live better and to improve the overall quality of life while undergoing treatment. Alyson adopted all aspects of the new Block Center program and began a third chemo cocktail. A short time thereafter, a targeted radiation treatment regimen was added to address swelling in her right leg.

Due to the aggressive nature of Alyson's cancer, she was never able to take full advantage of the Block Center's specialized program. In less than six months, it had spread from her reproductive system to her liver and lungs. We were preparing to try a fourth, and different, chemo cocktail recommendation, when we learned that the cancer had spread to the brain.

Alyson also attacked cancer with a warriorlike mindset, relying heavily on the qualities that led to her success in the water—as a competitive sprinter in the 50 race—hard work, dedication, determination, and an intense will to win. Alyson passed on Thursday, November 15, 2012, and her spirit also lives on through me and Simon the Cat.

This book is a tribute to their battles—their courage, grace, and all the ways in which they stood up to the enemy! In chapter 9, I included Coach Lombardi's clarification comments on his famous "winning" quote and I believe it's worth repeating. Coach Lombardi said, *"What I believe is, if you go out on a football field, or any endeavor in life, and you leave every fiber of what you have on the field, then you've won."* Max and Alyson fought this enemy every day and never backed down, and for that, they are the ultimate warriors and winners!

It is said that one never really gets over losses of the magnitude I've experienced. I believe that you don't get over this type of loss but that you get through difficult times by focusing on one day or one play at a time. The harsh reality is life goes on with or without us, whether we like it or not. I can think of no better anthem to provide you with the right mindset to get through challenging times than Argent's "Hold Your Head Up":

> *And if it's bad, don't let it get you down, you can take it.*
> *And if it hurts, don't let them see you cry, you can make it.*
> *Hold your head up, hold your head up,*
> *Hold your head up, hold your head high.*

I believe that there is good in all things, even in the loss of a loved one. In this case, our earthly loss, while painful, is their heavenly gain. I also believe that if you look closely, you can see what I refer to as signs, reinforcing this point. I'd like to leave you with an example of one such sign that occurred in my life that gives me cause for optimism about the future.

Green Light

It was an early Friday morning in December, and I was driving for the last time to my mother's house. The plan was to take the soon-to-be new owners through the house for a final walk-through and then go to their attorney's office to sign all of the closing-related documents. It was still hard to believe that a year had ended for me and Simon the Cat since Alyson passed, and two years for Max, and now we were selling her house, the family gathering place.

On this day, I took a different route from my house so that I could find the attorney's office prior to the closing. In the back of my mind, I was thinking about the importance of ending the book and this chapter of my life in a positive light, as well as providing readers with a sense of optimism for the future. As I turned off the side street onto the main street, I looked down the road, and as far as I could see, the traffic signals were all green. There must have been six or seven green lights directing me to Max's house, and then it hit me. The sign or message being given to me could not have been any more obvious. Simply put, you have the green light going forward with the next chapter of your life.

And just like in every other instance when I needed something for the book, it was given to me—this time in the form of green traffic lights as far as the eye could see, lighting the path to my mother's house and my future. A sense of calm came over me, and I smiled. What a great feeling and a truly liberating experience!

"And in the end, the love you take, is equal to the love, you make."
—Written by John Lennon and Paul McCartney
(the last song recorded collectively by all four of The Beatles)

ACKNOWLEDGMENTS

Max and Alyson were extraordinary women. Each of them had literally "an army" of supporters that were with them every step of the way. I want to thank this special group of individuals for their many acts of kindness and prayers during our greatest time of need. This group included family members, longtime friends, neighbors, classmates, work colleagues, church parishioners, and fellow cancer patients. Alyson also received an incredible amount of love and support from the Central PA swimming community, including the West Shore Y swimming coaching staff, swimmers, parents, longtime coaching buddy and good friend Coach Derrick Clemmer, and her Central Penn Masters teammates.

Max and Alyson were blessed with an exceptional group of highly skilled healthcare professionals—warriors in their own right—who cared for them and worked tirelessly on the frontlines every day of our battles. Our family was extremely thankful for the personal care we received from the following individuals and organizations: the PinnacleHealth Harrisburg Hospital emergency room medical team led by Ruchi Dash, MD; neurosurgeons Moksha Ranasinghe, MD and Hayden Boyce, MD; cardiovascular and thoracic surgery unit led by Troy Moritz, DO, FACOS; PinnacleHealth Helen M. Simpson Rehabilitation Hospital's nursing staff and physical/occupational therapy staff; and the PinnacleHealth Regional Cancer Center team led by Brij Sood, MD; specialists Warren Sewall, MD and Roy Williams, MD; and a truly special group of nursing and support staff. Other specialists included the Andrews & Patel Associates' team of oncologists; Kathryn Peroutka, MD; Anna Strickland of the NavigateCancer Foundation; Marianne Robleski of EmergingMed; and Jeanne Gutierrez of Target Now. The Block Center (Integrative

Cancer Treatment)—led by Keith I. Block, MD and his team of doctors, physician assistants, treatment specialists, and support staff—was also instrumental. I also want to thank the members of the Penn State Milton S. Hershey Medical Center Obstetrics and Gynecology care team led by Joshua P. Kesterson, MD.

We were fortunate to have two personal friends that were also highly skilled doctors: Matt Mumber, MD, a radiation oncologist and author that resides at the Harbin Clinic, Georgia, and Audrey Krosnowski, MD, a radiologist specializing in diagnostic radiology from the Health Image at South Denver, Englewood, Colorado. It gave us peace of mind to know that we could receive an honest assessment of each health challenge, including the potential likelihood of all outcomes, at every step in the journey.

I want to thank the lead scientist for the IBM Research and Watson technology program—Dr. (Marty) Kohn, MS, MD, FACEP, FACPE, Chief Medical Scientist, Care Delivery Systems IBM Research—for his act of compassion in responding to a son's desperate inquiry to use IBM's leading-edge medical computer system, "Watson," to help his mother's doctors find a cure for her medical condition. While the technology was in the early stages of development at the time, December 2011, I have no doubt that in the very near future it will be an invaluable tool and resource for not only families confronting challenging health conditions but also the medical professionals tasked with providing their care.

The following special friendships were sources of strength and encouragement for me during both battles with cancer and the eventual writing of this book: Brian and Judy Bullock; Joe, Jane, Alyson, and Nicholas Tamanini; Bill Matson; Scott and Tina Johnson; Andy and Brie Krosnowski; Steve Hare; Tom Reed; John Krosnowski; Gregg and Michelle Sheibley; Ed Zionkofski; Tom Nye; Will Mowrey; Brandt Cook; Coach Derrick and Amy Clemmer; John and Mary Flynn; Shawn Lawton; Edward Tonnesen; Jay Lichtel; Ryan Priest; Jay Pizoli; Jeff Martin; Debra Pierson; Steve Muschlitz; Justine Evelyn; John Nugent; Dennis Pacy; Dennis and Andrew Zimmerman; Glenn Swan; Jon Yuninger; Larry Fox; Beth Burn; Bryan Withington; Mike Curley; David Hankins; and my sister, Tina.

And, these individuals also had the distinction of being members of my review and editing team: Pete Weaver, aunt Joan Graham, Judy Hollander, Rick Pierce, Linda Mowrey, Jeff Lichtel, Harry "Four" Chapman IV, Dr. Lee Morand, Ed Coffey, and Deborah Maguire.

As for the actual writing of this book, I would first like to thank my good friend Matt Mumber, MD and his wife Laura. Matt and Laura had just been through the process of writing and publishing his first book, *Sustainable Wellness: An Integrative Approach to Transform Your Mind, Body, and Spirit*, when I asked him to read a first draft. His encouragement led me to seek out a developmental editor. It took some time, but I was so fortunate to find Wendy Lazear, a talented editor extraordinaire without whom this book would not have been possible. Wendy and I developed an immediate personal connection and writing chemistry. This special writing relationship allowed us to take a raw story and transform it into the basis for the book you are holding in your hands. Thankfully, Wendy also came back on board at the end of the project to bring the book to completion.

With Cathy Kessler, my gifted copyeditor and proofreader, I also developed an instant writing chemistry. We worked for the better part of six months on the logical flow of the copy, along with filling in any missing pieces of information. Cathy provided me with the right blend of encouragement and a sense of urgency to ensure that I accomplished my personal goal of completing this book.

Thanks to Mike Lazear, owner of White Sands Web, LLC, specialists in using the latest web technologies to create a unique online presence for their clients, for building a custom website to facilitate the online marketing and promotion of the book. Thanks also goes to Bruce Baker, Claire Simms, and the Page Publishing, Inc. support staff for taking on this project and dedicating the time and effort required to make this book a reality.

I want to recognize the following special acts of kindness: Gretchen Wolford for sharing the treatment journey and experiences of her husband (Chester); PinnacleHealth Spiritual Care support staff and Pastor Donald Slaybaugh, Jr. for their calming influence and message of hope; John Krosnowski and his family for contributing to Alyson's travel costs to receive specialized treatments by the Block Center; Bill Matson for showing up at the hospital twice without a call to help me through two of the toughest nights of my life; Jim

Cooper for his words of wisdom to stay true to my story and myself at a crucial time in the writing process; Joe Green for his insights and advice on how to navigate the healthcare system to ensure the highest level of care for my mother and wife; Steve McGarvey for his time and effort to create the initial cover art for the book; and Gregg Sheibley for the design and creation of the book cover. I also want to thank the following individuals for providing me with valuable feedback on the draft manuscript, as well as a personal quote for the cover: Lee W. Morand, Psy. D.; Ruchi Dash, MD; Kathryn Peroutka, MD; Anne Wagoner; Deborah Maguire; Paul Y. Song, MD; Pete Weaver; Tina Johnson; and Roy A. Williams, MD.

My family was very appreciative of the encouragement and support Max received from longtime neighbors and friends Carolyn and Rich Hubert, Dot and Ray Yeich, Linda and Robert "Skip" Geary, and Sharon and Ann Marie Johnson. Alyson and I were also very grateful for the support she received from our neighbors: Edie McDonald, Karen and Ray Roberts, Terry Bennett, Lynn and Joe Gaffney, Diane and John Butina, and Laura and Joe Marcucci.

I want to thank the following families for including me in their holiday plans and special family occasions: the Bullock family, the Wrabel family, the Hart family, the Tamanini family, the Johnson family, the Matson family, the Krosnowski family, and the Hoover family. The many acts of kindness by these very special families have helped me to experience, once again, the joy and happiness associated with family get-togethers and holiday celebrations.

Last, but not least, I want to thank my aunt Bonnie (Marty) for her energy, encouragement, and enthusiasm in providing me with a sounding board for ideas and a second set of proofreading eyes throughout the writing of this book; Simon the Cat for being my little buddy and helping me to get through the last year; and my mother and best friend for her painstaking efforts to help me refine my writing skills over the last twenty years so that it would one day be possible for me to write a book.

HONORABLE MENTION

I am extremely blessed to have had some very extraordinary individuals in my life. I want to take this opportunity to recognize and thank these special human beings for helping me to become the person I am today: my grandparents, the most kindhearted people I have ever met that showed me that prosperity is measured by more than the size of your bank account; Robert "Skip" Geary, the father of a good friend growing up, neighbor, and baseball coach on the importance of doing things "the right" way; Richard Smith, my fifth-grade teacher that instilled in me that the actions of a leader can have a positive or negative influence on others; Coach Harry Chapman III, my high-school football coach that used football to teach the importance of work ethic, sacrifice for the team, persistence and perseverance, and overcoming adversity if you want to succeed in football and life; Rich Lichtel, a teacher, football coach, and mentor on the importance of helping others to succeed and to have passion and enthusiasm for whatever you choose to do in life; Kenneth Reeher, the father of a high-school friend on what it means to be a professional and exude professionalism; Gary Lurie, an IBM colleague on the importance of delivering superior customer service while maintaining business profitability; Steve Wagoner, my newest friend on the power and strength of special friendships; and last, but not least, my father, Frank Jr., on striving for excellence in everything that you do.

ABOUT THE AUTHOR

Frank Antonicelli, III is a management consultant and founder of Public Safety Information Consulting, Inc. (PSIC), a technology-based consulting and services company. Prior to forming PSIC, Frank was a public sector marketing representative and systems integration specialist for IBM. He received his Bachelor of Science degree from Bloomsburg University of Pennsylvania and is a member of the Delta Omega Chi (DOC) Fraternity. Frank graduated from Cumberland Valley High School where he played football for the legendary Pennsylvania coach Harry C. Chapman III.

Frank enjoys spending time with family, friends, and Simon the Cat; restoring and driving classic Corvettes; physical fitness training and sports in general; coaching; playing golf; working in the yard; feeding the birds and rabbits; listening to music; writing poetry; and following the driver of the National Guard #88 Chevrolet—Dale Earnhardt Jr. Also, Frank is currently completing a two-year home remodeling project that combines the old charm and character of the home's 1920s architecture with modern living conveniences to create an updated two-story brick house.

Frank is also a founding member of the Rich Lichtel Memorial Fund, www.richlichtel.org.

CPSIA information can be obtained at www.ICGtesting.com
Printed in the USA
BVOW02*1424020616

450370BV00001B/1/P